THE
FLAT TUMMY
BLUEPRINT

Simple Strategies for a Leaner Midsection

Kayla S. Brigman

Dedication

This book is dedicated to my family and friends, who have always supported me and encouraged me to pursue my passion for health and wellness. Your love and support have been my source of strength and inspiration throughout this journey.

To my readers, who have entrusted me with the responsibility of helping them achieve their fitness goals. Your commitment to improving your health has motivated me to create this blueprint, and I hope it serves as a valuable resource on your journey to a healthier lifestyle.

And finally, to all the fitness professionals and experts who have generously shared their knowledge and expertise with me. Your contributions have been invaluable in shaping the content of this book, and I am deeply grateful for your support.

Thank you all for being a part of this journey.

Foreword

As a fitness expert, I have seen countless individuals struggle to achieve a leaner midsection, despite their best efforts. That's why I am thrilled to see a book like *"The Flat Tummy Blueprint"* enter the market, providing simple and effective strategies to help individuals achieve their fitness goals.

In this book, the author presents a comprehensive approach to achieving a flat tummy, including tips on nutrition, exercise, mindset, and lifestyle habits. The strategies presented in this book are backed by scientific research and the author's extensive experience in the field of fitness.

What I appreciate most about this book is its emphasis on sustainable lifestyle changes rather than quick-fix solutions. The author understands that achieving and maintaining a leaner midsection requires a holistic approach, and this book provides a roadmap to help readers make lasting changes.

Whether you are just starting on your fitness journey or are a seasoned athlete, *"The Flat Tummy Blueprint"* is an invaluable resource that can help you achieve your goals. I highly recommend this book to anyone looking to improve their health and fitness.

– Arlene van Roosmalen

Table of Contents

Introduction

This book is for those who are currently feeling self-conscious about their tummies. Do you wish you could confidently show off your midsection in any outfit? Well, you're in the right place! In this book, we will provide you with a step-by-step guide to achieving a flat tummy.

We know that losing weight and getting fit can be overwhelming, which is why we've designed this book to be as simple and straightforward as possible. You won't find any gimmicks or fad diets here – just proven, science-backed strategies that will help you shed excess belly fat and tone up your midsection.

Throughout this book, we'll cover topics such as nutrition, exercise, and lifestyle habits that can impact your belly fat. We'll also provide you with practical tips and tools to help you stay on track and achieve your flat tummy goals.

Whether you're a beginner or an experienced fitness enthusiast, we believe that anyone can benefit from the information in this book. So if you're ready to get started, let's dive in and begin your journey to a leaner, healthier midsection!

Chapter 1

Understanding the Causes of Belly Fat and How to Measure Your Progress

Belly fat, abdominal fat or obesity is a common concern. Not only can it be unsightly, but it can also have profound health implications. In this chapter, we'll explore the causes of belly fat, the risks associated with excess abdominal fat, and how to measure your progress as you work towards a flat tummy.

What Causes Belly Fat?

Several factors can contribute to excess abdominal fat, including:

- ***Poor diet:***

Consuming an unhealthy diet high in refined carbs, added sugars, and unhealthy fats can lead to weight gain, particularly in the abdominal area.

- ***Lack of physical activity:***

Leading a sedentary lifestyle can contribute to weight gain, including abdominal fat.

- ***Stress:***

Chronic stress can lead to the release of the hormone cortisol, which has been linked to weight gain, particularly in the abdominal area.

- ***Aging:***

As we age, our metabolism slows down, making gaining weight, including abdominal fat, easier.

- **Genetics:**

Some people may be more prone to carrying excess weight in their abdominal area due to genetic factors.

What Are The Risks Associated With Belly Fat?

Excess abdominal fat (fat that surrounds your organs) can increase the risk of several severe health conditions, including:

- **Heart disease:**

Abdominal fat has been linked to an increased risk of heart disease and stroke.

- **Diabetes:**

Excess abdominal fat can increase the risk of developing type 2 diabetes.

- **Certain cancers:**

Abdominal fat has been linked to an increased risk of certain types of cancer, including colon, breast, and endometrial cancer.

- **Metabolic syndrome:**

Excess abdominal fat is often accompanied by other risk factors for metabolic syndrome, a group of conditions that increase the risk of heart disease, diabetes, and stroke.

How Do I Measure My Progress?

As you work towards a flat tummy, tracking your progress is crucial to stay motivated and on track. There are several ways to measure your progress, including:

- **Waist measurement:**

Measuring your waist at its narrowest point can give you an indication of your abdominal fat. A waist measurement of more than 35 inches for women or 40 inches for men is considered a risk factor for health problems.

- ***Body mass index (BMI):***

This measure considers your weight and height to determine your overall body fat percentage. While it's not a perfect measure, a BMI of 25 or higher is considered overweight, while a BMI of 30 or higher is considered obese.

- ***Before-and-after photos:***

Taking photos of yourself at the beginning of your journey and comparing them to those taken later can give you a visual representation of your progress.

- ***Other measurements:***

In addition to waist measurement and BMI, you can also measure other areas of your body, such as your hips and thighs, to track your progress.

By understanding the causes of belly fat, the risks associated with excess abdominal fat, and how to measure your progress, you'll be well on your way to achieving a flat tummy.

Understanding the Science of a Leaner Midsection

Understanding the science of a leaner midsection is critical to achieving your goals for a flatter tummy. While many factors, such as diet, exercise, and lifestyle habits, can contribute to a slimmer midsection, the underlying science is complex and multifaceted.

One of the critical factors in achieving a leaner midsection is reducing overall body fat. Fat cells accumulate in different body parts depending on genetic and hormonal factors, but the abdominal region is a common area where fat can accumulate. When we consume more calories than our bodies can burn, the excess energy is stored in fat cells throughout the body, including the abdominal region.

Reducing body fat is vital for achieving a flatter tummy, but it is not just about doing endless ab exercises. Targeted ab exercises can help tone and strengthen your core muscles, but they won't necessarily reduce the amount of fat stored in your abdominal region.

To achieve a leaner midsection, you must focus on overall body composition changes through cardiovascular exercise, strength training, and a healthy diet.

Cardiovascular exercises like running, cycling, or swimming can help burn calories and boost metabolism, leading to overall fat loss. On the other hand, strength training can help build lean muscle mass, increasing metabolism and leading to long-term fat loss.

A healthy diet, including plenty of fruits and vegetables, lean protein, and healthy fats, can create a calorie deficit and promote overall body composition changes.

It's also important to note that the amount of abdominal fat you have can be influenced by various other factors, such as genetics, hormones, and age. For example, women tend to store more fat in their abdominal region than men due to hormonal differences.

Additionally, our metabolism naturally slows down as we age, making it harder to lose weight and maintain a lean midsection.

Incorporating healthy habits, such as getting enough sleep, managing stress levels, and avoiding excessive alcohol consumption, can also contribute to a leaner midsection.

Lack of sleep and high-stress levels can increase cortisol levels, a hormone that promotes fat storage in the abdominal region. Additionally, excessive alcohol consumption can increase calorie intake and bloating, making it harder to achieve a flatter tummy.

In summary, achieving a leaner midsection is not just about doing endless crunches or following fad diets. It's about understanding the complex interactions between your diet, exercise, and lifestyle habits and making sustainable changes to promote overall body composition changes.

By reducing overall body fat through cardiovascular exercise, strength training, and a healthy diet and incorporating healthy habits into your daily routine, you can achieve your goals for a flatter tummy.

In the next chapter, we'll delve into the importance of nutrition for a flat tummy.

Chapter 2

The Importance of Nutrition for a Flat Tummy

Proper nutrition is an essential component of achieving and maintaining a flat tummy. In this chapter, we'll explore nutrition's role in weight loss and how to make healthy food choices to support your flat tummy goals.

The Role of Nutrition in Weight Loss

When it comes to losing weight and getting fit, it's important to remember that calories matter. To lose weight, you must create a calorie deficit, which means burning more calories than you consume. While exercise is an integral part of the equation, what you eat significantly impacts your weight loss efforts.

Eating a healthy, balanced diet can help you lose weight, including belly fat, by providing your body with the nutrients it needs to function correctly. This includes:

1. **Protein:**

Protein helps build and repair tissues and helps you feel full and satisfied, which can aid in weight loss. Good protein sources include *lean meats, poultry, fish, eggs, beans,* and *legumes.*

2. **Fiber:**

The fiber in whole grains can help your body feel full and satisfied, which can reduce your cravings and prevent overeating. Good sources of fiber include beans, whole grains, fruits, and vegetables.

3. **Healthy fats:**

Despite the negative reputation that fats have had in the past, certain types of fat are good for you and can help with weight loss. These include:

- Monounsaturated fats (found in olive oil, nuts, and avocados).
- Polyunsaturated fats (found in vegetable oils and fatty fish).

4. **Complex carbs:**

Complex carbs, instead of refined carbs, provide your body with sustained energy and are an essential source of nutrients. Good sources of complex carbs include whole grains, fruits, vegetables, and legumes.

Making Healthy Food Choices

To support your flat tummy goals, you must make healthy food choices. Here are some essential tips for making healthy food choices:

- ***Focus on whole, unprocessed foods:***

Choose foods as close to their natural state as possible, such as fruits, vegetables, whole grains, and lean proteins.

- ***Limit added sugars and unhealthy fats:***

Foods high in added sugars and unhealthy fats, such as fried foods and processed snacks, can contribute to weight gain, particularly in the abdominal area.

- ***Portion control:***

It's essential to pay attention to portion sizes to avoid overeating. Use measuring cups or a food scale to consume appropriate portions.

- ***Plan ahead:***

Planning your meals and snacks can help you stay on track and make healthy food choices.

By focusing on proper nutrition and healthy food choices, you'll be well on your way to achieving a flat tummy. The following section will delve into specific foods that can help burn belly fat.

The Best Foods for Burning Belly Fat

While calorie control and proper nutrition are essential for losing weight, including belly fat, certain foods may have a more pronounced effect on abdominal fat. This chapter will explore some of the best foods for burning belly fat and how to incorporate them into your diet.

1. **Avocados:**

These creamy, nutritious fruits are high in monounsaturated fats, which have been shown to help reduce belly fat. They're also a good source of fiber, which can help you feel full and satisfied. Add sliced avocado to sandwiches, salads, or toast, or use mashed avocado to spread on sandwiches or wraps.

2. **Nuts and seeds:**

Nuts and seeds are good sources of protein, fiber, and healthy fats, which can help with weight loss. Studies have shown that people who consume nuts tend to have less belly fat than those who don't.

Add a small handful of nuts or seeds to your meals or snacks, or use nut or seed butter as a spread on toast or as a dip for fruits and vegetables.

3. **Berries:**

Berries are high in fiber and antioxidants, which can help with weight loss and reduce inflammation in the body. Some studies have shown that people who consume more berries tend to have less belly fat than those who don't.

Try adding a handful of berries to your breakfast oatmeal or yogurt, or use them as a topping for salads or desserts.

4. **Green tea:**

Green tea is high in antioxidants and has been shown to increase metabolism and fat oxidation, which can help with weight loss, including belly fat. Try swapping out your regular coffee or tea for green tea, or add a supplement to your daily routine.

5. *Turmeric:*

This spice is high in curcumin, a compound shown to reduce inflammation and help with weight loss. Add turmeric to your meals or drinks, or try a turmeric supplement.

6. *Leafy greens:*

Leafy greens, such as spinach, kale, and broccoli, are low in calories and fiber, which can help with weight loss. They're also high in antioxidants and other nutrients supporting overall health. You can try adding a serving of leafy greens to your meals or smoothies.

By incorporating these belly fat-burning foods into your diet, you'll be on your way to a leaner, healthier midsection. Remember, however, that weight loss is about more than specific foods – focusing on proper nutrition and calorie control is also essential.

Strategies for Incorporating Healthy Habits into Your Daily Routine

This section will explore practical tips and techniques for incorporating healthy habits into your daily routine to support a leaner midsection.

Hydration

First and foremost, let's talk about hydration. Drinking enough water is crucial for maintaining a healthy weight and promoting a leaner midsection. When dehydrated, your body may retain moisture, leading to bloating and puffiness. Aim to drink at least eight glasses of water daily, and more if you're exercising or in hot weather.

Fiber

Next, let's talk about fiber. Bloating and digestion can be regulated by eating food high in fiber, like whole grains, vegetables, and fruits. Fiber can also help you feel fuller for longer, reducing the likelihood of overeating or snacking on unhealthy foods. Aim to include a variety of high-fiber foods in your diet, and consider taking a fiber supplement if you need more throughout your diet.

Protein

Incorporating protein into your diet is also crucial for supporting a leaner midsection. Protein helps build and repair muscles, increasing metabolism and promoting fat loss. Aim to include a source of protein in each meal, such as chicken, fish, tofu, or beans.

Mindful Eating Habits

In addition to focusing on specific nutrients, it's important to practice mindful eating habits. Eat slowly and without interruptions while paying attention to your body's hunger and fullness signs. Doing so can reduce the likelihood of overeating and promote a healthier relationship with food.

Managing Stress Levels

Another critical aspect of supporting a leaner midsection is managing stress levels. High-stress levels can lead to increased levels of cortisol, a hormone that promotes fat storage in the abdominal region.

Incorporating stress-reducing practices into your daily routine, such as meditation, yoga, or deep breathing, can help mitigate these effects.

Sleep

Finally, getting enough sleep is crucial for achieving a leaner midsection. Lack of sleep can lead to increased cortisol and insulin resistance levels, making it harder to lose weight and maintain a healthy weight. Aim to get 7-9 hours of sleep per night and prioritize a consistent sleep schedule.

Nutrition for a Flat Tummy: The Best Foods to Eat and Avoid

This section will discuss the best foods to eat and avoid supporting a flat tummy. First, let's talk about the best foods to eat. A diet rich in whole, nutrient-dense foods supports a flat stomach. These foods include:

1. **Leafy greens:**

Leafy greens, such as collard greens, kale, and spinach, are packed with fiber, minerals, and vitamins. They are also low in calories, making them a fantastic weight-loss choice.

2. Lean protein:

Protein is essential for building and repairing muscles, which can help increase metabolism and promote fat loss. Good lean protein sources include chicken, turkey, fish, tofu, and legumes.

3. Whole grains:

Whole grains, such as quinoa, brown rice, and whole wheat bread, are fiber-rich, which can help regulate digestion and reduce bloating.

4. Fruits and vegetables:

Fruits and vegetables are packed with minerals, vitamins, and fiber. They are also low in calories, making them a huge weight-loss choice.

5. Nuts and seeds:

Nuts and seeds are rich in healthy fats, protein, and fiber, which can help you feel fuller for longer.

Foods to Avoid

Now let's discuss the foods to avoid if you want a flat tummy. These include:

1. *Processed foods:*

Processed food is typically loaded with calories, unhealthy fats, and sugar, and the nutrients are often lacking. As a result, weight gain and bloating can occur as a result of them.

2. *Sugar-sweetened beverages:*

Sugar-sweetened beverages, such as soda and fruit juice, are high in sugar and calories and can contribute to weight gain.

3. *Fried foods:*

Fried foods are often high in unhealthy fats and calories and can contribute to weight gain and inflammation.

4. Alcohol:

Alcohol is high in calories and can contribute to weight gain and bloating.

5. High-sodium foods:

High-sodium foods like processed meats and canned soups can contribute to bloating and water retention.

In conclusion, a diet rich in whole, nutrient-dense foods is essential for supporting a flat tummy. This includes leafy greens, lean protein, whole grains, fruits and vegetables, and nuts and seeds.

To support a flat tummy, you must avoid processed foods, sugar-sweetened beverages, fried foods, alcohol, and high-sodium foods. By making these dietary changes, you can support your goals for a flatter tummy and overall improved health.

In the next chapter, we'll delve into exercise's role in achieving a flat tummy.

Chapter 3

The Role of Exercise in Achieving a Flat Tummy

Exercise is an essential component of achieving and maintaining a flat tummy. In this chapter, we'll explore the different types of exercise that can help you burn belly fat and how to create an effective exercise plan.

The Types of Exercise That Can Help You Burn Belly Fat

Various kinds of exercise can help you burn belly fat, including:

- *Cardio:*

Cardio exercises, such as running, cycling, and swimming, increase your heart rate and burn calories, which can help with weight loss, including belly fat.

- *Strength training:*

Strength training exercises, such as weight lifting, can help you build muscle, which can increase your metabolism and help you burn more calories throughout the day.

- *High-intensity interval training (HIIT):*

HIIT workouts involve short bursts of intense exercise followed by periods of rest. These workouts can be very effective for burning fat, including belly fat.

Creating an Effective Exercise Plan

To get the most out of your exercise routine, creating an effective plan that works for you is crucial. Here are some tips for creating an effective exercise plan:

- ***Set specific goals:***

Determine what you want to achieve with your exercise routine and make specific, measurable goals. For example, you might aim to lose weight or fit into a particular clothing size.

- ***Make a schedule:***

Plan out when you'll exercise and stick to it. Consider your work schedule, family commitments, and energy levels when creating your schedule.

- ***Choose exercises you enjoy:***

Choosing exercises you enjoy is essential, as this will make it more likely that you'll stick with your routine. If you hate running, for example, consider trying a different form of cardio, such as cycling or swimming.

- **Be consistent:**

Consistency is critical when it comes to exercise. Aim to exercise regularly rather than in sporadic bursts of activity.

- **Vary your workouts:**

Mixing up your workouts helps keep you motivated and prevents boredom. Try incorporating different types of exercise, such as cardio, strength training, and HIIT, into your routine.

By incorporating exercise into your routine and creating an effective plan, you'll be well on your way to achieving a flat tummy. In the next chapter, we'll delve into the specific benefits of cardio exercise for burning belly fat.

Cardio for Belly Fat Loss: Options and Tips

Cardio exercise is integral to any weight loss plan, including burning belly fat. In this chapter, we'll explore the benefits of cardio for belly fat loss and provide some tips for getting the most out of your cardio workouts.

The Benefits of Cardio for Belly Fat Loss

Cardio exercises like running, cycling, and swimming can effectively burn belly fat because they increase your heart rate and burn calories. Some of the specific benefits of cardio for belly fat loss include:

- ***Increased metabolism:***

Cardio can help to boost your metabolism, which can help you burn more calories throughout the day.

- ***Improved cardiovascular health:***

Cardio exercises can improve cardiovascular health by strengthening your heart and increasing blood flow.

- ***Stress reduction:***

Cardio can help reduce stress and improve your mood by releasing endorphins, chemicals that act as natural painkillers and mood elevators.

Tips for Getting the Most Out Of Your Cardio Workouts

To get the most out of your cardio workouts, try incorporating the following tips:

- ***Warm up and cool down:***

Start your workouts with a 5-10 minute warm-up to prepare your muscles and joints for exercise, and end with a cool-down to help your body recover.

- ***Vary your intensity:***

To keep your workouts challenging and prevent boredom, try alternating between high-intensity intervals and lower-intensity recovery periods.

- ***Mix up your workouts:***

In addition to varying your intensity, try incorporating different types of cardio into your routine, such as running, cycling, and swimming.

- ***Wear the right gear:***

Invest in a good pair of running or cycling shoes to help prevent injury and improve your performance.

- ***Stay hydrated:***

Ensure you drink plenty of water before, during, and after your workouts to stay hydrated and help your body perform at its best.

By incorporating cardio into your routine and following these tips, you'll be well on your way to burning belly fat and improving your overall health.

Exercise Strategies for a Flat Tummy: Targeting Your Abs and Core

In this section, we'll discuss the importance of regular exercise for achieving a flat tummy. Exercise is a critical component when it comes to getting a leaner midsection.

Not only can exercise help burn calories and reduce body fat, but it can also help build muscle and improve posture, leading to a flatter tummy.

Let's take a closer look at some of the best exercises for a flat tummy:

1. **Cardiovascular exercise:**

Cardiovascular exercises like running, cycling, or swimming can help burn calories and reduce body fat, which is vital for achieving a flatter tummy. Aim for at least 30 minutes of cardiovascular exercise most days of the week.

2. **Strength training:**

Strength training, such as weightlifting or bodyweight exercises, can help build muscle, increase metabolism and promote fat loss. Focus on exercises that target the core, such as planks, crunches, and Russian twists.

3. **Pilates:**

Pilates is a low-impact exercise focusing on core strength, flexibility, and posture. Many Pilates exercises are specifically designed to target the core muscles, making it an excellent choice for achieving a flatter tummy.

4. Yoga:

Like Pilates, yoga is a low-impact exercise that can help improve posture, flexibility, and core strength. Many yoga poses, such as the plank and boat pose, are also great for targeting the core muscles.

In addition to these exercises, it's also important to incorporate activities that promote overall movement, such as walking, hiking, or dancing. These activities can help burn calories and improve overall health, contributing to a flatter tummy.

When it comes to exercise for a flat tummy, consistency is key. Aim for at least 30 minutes of exercise most days of the week, and try to incorporate a mix of cardiovascular exercise, strength training, and low-impact activities like Pilates and yoga.

In conclusion, regular exercise is essential for achieving a flat tummy. Cardiovascular exercise, strength training, Pilates, and yoga are all great options for targeting the core muscles and promoting fat loss. By making exercise a regular part of your routine, you can support your goals for a leaner midsection and improved overall health.

In the next chapter, we'll delve into the benefits of strength training for a flat tummy.

Chapter 4

Strength Training for a Strong, Toned Midsection

In addition to cardio, strength training is an integral part of any weight loss plan, including achieving a flat tummy. In this chapter, we'll explore the benefits of strength training for a flat tummy and provide some tips for incorporating it into your routine.

The Benefits of Strength Training For a Flat Tummy

Strength training exercises, such as weight lifting and bodyweight exercises, can be practical for burning belly fat because they build muscle, which can increase your metabolism and help you burn more calories throughout the day. Some of the specific benefits of strength training for a flat tummy include the following:

- ***Increased muscle mass***: Strength training can help you build muscle mass, which can help to tone and define your midsection.

- ***Improved posture***: Strength training can help improve your posture, making your tummy appear flatter and more toned.

- ***Increased bone density***: Strength training can help increase bone density, reducing the risk of osteoporosis and other bone-related conditions.

Tips for Incorporating Strength Training Into Your Routine

To get the most out of your strength training workouts, try incorporating the following tips:

1. ***Start with bodyweight exercises:***

If you're new to strength training, start with bodyweight exercises, such as push-ups, squats, and lunges, to build a foundation of strength.

2. ***Gradually increase the weight:***

As you become more comfortable with strength training, gradually increase the weight or resistance to challenge your muscles and continue to build strength.

3. ***Vary your workouts:***

Mixing up your strength training workouts helps keep you motivated and prevents boredom. Try incorporating different types of exercises, such as weight lifting, bodyweight exercises, and resistance bands, into your routine.

4. *Use proper form:*

It's essential to use proper form when training to avoid injury and ensure you're targeting the correct muscles. Consider working with a personal trainer or consulting a fitness professional to ensure you use the proper form.

5. *Rest and recover:*

Allowing your muscles time to rest and recover between strength training sessions is essential. Take a 48-hour break between strength training workouts to allow your muscles to recover.

By incorporating strength training into your routine and following these tips, you'll be well on your way to a strong, toned midsection. In the next section, we'll delve into the benefits of high-intensity interval training (HIIT) for burning belly fat.

High-Intensity Interval Training (HIIT) for a Flat Tummy

High-intensity interval training (HIIT) is a type of exercise involving short bursts of intense activity followed by rest periods. HIIT workouts can be very effective for burning belly fat and improving overall fitness. In this chapter, we'll explore the benefits of HIIT for burning belly fat and provide some tips for incorporating it into your routine.

The Benefits of High-Intensity Interval Training (HIIT) for Burning Belly Fat

HIIT workouts can be particularly effective for burning belly fat because they increase your heart rate and metabolism and can be done in a shorter amount of time compared to other types of workouts. Some of the specific benefits of HIIT for burning belly fat include:

- ***Increased fat loss***: HIIT workouts can help increase fat loss, including belly fat, due to the high-intensity workouts.

- ***Improved cardiovascular fitness***: HIIT workouts can improve your cardiovascular fitness by strengthening your heart and increasing blood flow.

- ***Increased metabolism***: HIIT workouts can boost your metabolism, which can help you burn more calories throughout the day.

Tips for Incorporating HIIT into Your Routine

To get the most out of your HIIT workouts, try incorporating the following tips:

1. ***Start with shorter intervals***:

If you're new to HIIT, start with shorter intervals of intense activity and gradually increase the length as you become more comfortable.

2. **Use proper form:**

Using proper form when doing HIIT is essential to avoid injury and ensure you get the most out of your workouts.

3. **Vary your workouts:**

Mixing up your HIIT workouts helps keep you motivated and prevents boredom. Try incorporating different types of exercises, such as running, cycling, and bodyweight exercises, into your routine.

4. **Allow for proper recovery:**

HIIT workouts are intense and physically demanding, so it's essential to allow proper recovery between sessions. Aim to give your body 48 hours of rest between HIIT workouts.

5. ***Incorporate other forms of exercise:***

While HIIT can be an effective form of exercise for burning belly fat, it's crucial to incorporate other forms of exercise into your routine, such as strength training and cardio. Including other forms of exercise can help to create a well-rounded fitness plan and prevent overtraining.

By incorporating HIIT into your routine and following these tips, you'll be well on your way to burning belly fat and improving your overall fitness. In the next chapter, we'll delve into the role of sleep in achieving a flat tummy.

The Need for Proper Hydration

In this section, we'll be discussing the importance of proper hydration for achieving a flat tummy. Many people don't realize that staying hydrated is essential for maintaining a healthy weight and gaining a flat tummy. When you don't drink enough water, your body can become dehydrated, leading to bloating and water retention. Dehydration can make your midsection appear larger and less defined.

Here are some tips for staying hydrated and promoting a flat tummy:

1. **Drink plenty of water:**

Aim for at least 8-10 glasses of water per day. Drinking water can help flush toxins from your body and reduce bloating.

2. **Limit alcohol and caffeine:**

Alcohol and caffeine can dehydrate your body, leading to bloating and water retention. Limit your intake of these beverages and choose water or herbal tea instead.

3. **Eat water-rich foods:**

Fruits and vegetables are excellent sources of water, which can help you stay hydrated and promote a flatter tummy. Some great options include cucumbers, watermelon, strawberries, and lettuce.

4. ***Avoid sugary drinks***:

Sugary drinks, such as soda and juice, can contribute to weight gain and bloating. Choose water or herbal tea instead.

5. ***Consider electrolyte drinks***:

If you're exercising or sweating heavily, electrolyte drinks can help replenish the fluids and minerals lost through sweat.

Staying hydrated can promote a healthier body weight and a flatter tummy. Drinking plenty of water, limiting alcohol and caffeine, eating water-rich foods, avoiding sugary drinks, and considering electrolyte drinks when needed can all help you achieve your hydration goals.

In addition to promoting a flatter tummy, proper hydration has many other benefits, including improved digestion, better skin health, and increased energy levels. So, prioritize hydration as part of your overall health and wellness routine.

Mindset and Motivation for a Flat Tummy: Staying on Track with Your Goals

This section will discuss the importance of mindset and motivation for achieving and maintaining a flat tummy. When making healthy lifestyle changes, such as eating a nutritious diet and exercising regularly, having a positive mindset and staying motivated are key.

Here are some tips for staying on track with your goals and achieving a flat tummy:

1. Set realistic goals:

It's essential to set goals that are achievable and realistic. Instead of aiming for a specific weight or dress size, focus on behaviors you can control, such as exercising regularly and eating a healthy diet.

2. Keep a positive mindset:

A positive mindset can make all the difference in sticking to your goals. Instead of focusing on what you can't have or do, focus on what you can do and how good it feels to take care of your body.

3. Find a support system:

Having a support system can help keep you motivated and accountable. Consider joining a fitness class, finding a workout buddy, or seeking support from a health coach or therapist.

4. **Track your progress:**

Keeping track of your progress can keep you motivated and help you see your progress. Consider taking measurements, tracking your workouts, or keeping a food diary.

5. **Celebrate your successes:**

Staying motivated and positive can be achieved by celebrating your successes, no matter how small they may be. Consider rewarding yourself with a non-food treat, such as a massage or new workout gear, when you reach a milestone.

6. **Practice self-care:**

Taking care of your mental and emotional health is as important as your physical health. Take time for yourself, practice self-compassion, and manage stress through activities like yoga, meditation, or deep breathing.

In conclusion, mindset and motivation are essential to achieving and maintaining a flat tummy. By setting realistic goals, keeping a positive attitude, finding a support system, tracking your progress, celebrating your successes, and practicing self-care, you can stay on track with your goals and achieve a healthier, leaner midsection.

Remember, minor changes can lead to significant results, so be patient, consistent, and motivated.

Chapter 5

The Importance of Sleep for a Flat Tummy

Getting enough quality sleep is an integral part of any weight loss plan, including achieving a flat tummy. In this chapter, we'll explore the role of sleep in weight loss and provide some tips for improving your sleep habits.

The Role of Sleep in Weight Loss

Sleep plays a crucial role in maintaining overall health and well-being and can also significantly impact weight loss efforts. Studies have shown that people who get enough sleep don't tend to have a higher risk of obesity, including abdominal obesity. Some of the ways that sleep can affect weight loss include:

- **Metabolism:**

Sleep plays a role in regulating metabolism, and inadequate sleep can disrupt the hormonal balance that regulates appetite and metabolism. This can make it more challenging to lose weight, including belly fat.

- **Hunger and appetite:**

Lack of sleep can increase hunger and appetite, particularly for high-fat and high-calorie foods.

- **Exercise performance:**

Adequate sleep is essential for optimal exercise performance. When well-rested, you'll be able to exercise harder and longer, which can help with weight loss.

Tips for Improving Your Sleep Habits

To get the most out of your sleep and support your weight loss efforts, try incorporating the following tips:

- ***Set a consistent sleep schedule:***

Aim to go to bed and wake up simultaneously every day, even on weekends, to establish a consistent sleep schedule.

- ***Create a sleep-friendly environment:***

Make sure that your bedroom is conducive to sleep by keeping it dark, quiet, and at a comfortable temperature.

- ***Avoid screens before bed:***

You should avoid screens at least an hour before going to sleep because screens emit blue light that interferes with melatonin production

- ***Relax before bed:***

Try to relax and wind down before bed by reading a book or taking a warm bath.

- ***Avoid caffeine and alcohol:***

Caffeine and alcohol can disrupt sleep, so avoid consuming them before bedtime.

By prioritizing sleep and improving your sleep habits, you'll be well on your way to achieving a flat tummy and overall good health.

The Benefits of Yoga for a Flat Tummy

Yoga is a centuries-old practice that combines physical postures, breathing techniques, and meditation to promote physical and mental well-being. In addition to its many other benefits, yoga can effectively achieve a flat tummy.

One of the primary benefits of yoga for a flat tummy is its ability to strengthen and tone the abdominal muscles. Many yoga poses, such as the plank, downward facing dog, and boat pose, engage the core muscles and help to build strength and definition in the midsection.

In addition to strengthening the muscles, these poses can also improve flexibility and mobility in the spine and hips, which can help to improve posture and make the tummy appear flatter.

In addition to its physical benefits, yoga can also help with weight loss and belly fat reduction. Yoga can increase flexibility and strength, which can help boost metabolism and burn calories.

Some studies have also shown that yoga can reduce stress and improve sleep, which can be factored into weight gain and difficulty losing weight, including belly fat.

To get the most out of your yoga practice for a flat tummy, consider incorporating the following tips:

- ***Put your focus on poses that engage your core:***

Incorporate a variety of yoga poses that engage the core muscles, such as plank, boat pose, and downward facing dog, into your practice.

- ***Practice regularly:***

To see the benefits of yoga for a flat tummy, aim to practice regularly, at least a few times a week.

- ***Incorporate other forms of exercise:***

While yoga is an effective way to strengthen and tone the core muscles, it's crucial to incorporate other forms of exercise, such as cardio and strength training, into your routine to create a well-rounded fitness plan.

- ***Listen to your body:***

It's essential to listen to your body and practice safely and comfortably. If you're new to yoga, consider starting with a beginner's class or working with a private instructor to ensure you use proper form and avoid injury.

By incorporating yoga into your routine and following these tips, you'll be well on your way to achieving a strong, toned, and flat tummy. In the next chapter, we'll delve into the role of nutrition in achieving a flat tummy.

Strength Training

This section will discuss the benefits of strength training for achieving a flat tummy. Many people believe cardio is the key to losing weight and getting a flat tummy, but strength training can be just as necessary.

Strength training can help you build lean muscle mass, which can boost your metabolism and help you burn more calories throughout the day. Additionally, strength training can help you tone and define your midsection muscles, which can help you achieve a flatter tummy.

Here are some tips for incorporating strength training into your workout routine:

1. *Focus on compound exercises:*

Compound exercises, such as squats, deadlifts, and bench presses, work multiple muscle groups at once, which can help you build strength and burn more calories. These exercises can also help you engage your core muscles, which can help you achieve a flatter tummy.

2. *Incorporate HIIT workouts:*

High-intensity interval training (HIIT) workouts can help you burn more calories and build strength in less time. These workouts typically involve short bursts of high-intensity exercise followed by rest periods.

3. Use resistance bands or weights:

Using resistance bands or weights can help you increase the resistance and challenge of your exercises, which can help you build strength and tone your muscles.

4. Don't forget about your abs:

While compound exercises can help you engage your core muscles, it's also important to include exercises explicitly targeting your abs, such as crunches and planks.

5. Give your muscles time to recover:

Giving your muscles time to recover after strength training workouts is essential. Aim to train each muscle group 2-3 times per week and allow at least one day of rest between workouts.

In addition to helping you achieve a flatter tummy, strength training has many other benefits for overall health, including improved bone density, better posture, and increased strength and endurance. So, prioritize strength training as part of your general fitness routine.

Remember, it's essential to consult with a healthcare professional before starting any new exercise program, especially if you have any underlying health conditions or injuries. Additionally, start with lighter weights or resistance bands and gradually increase the intensity and challenge of your workouts over time.

By focusing on compound exercises, incorporating HIIT workouts, using resistance bands or weights, targeting your abs, and allowing time for muscle recovery, you can build lean muscle mass, boost your metabolism, and achieve a healthier, slimmer midsection.

In conclusion, incorporating strength training into your workout routine can be a powerful tool for achieving a flatter tummy and overall health and wellness.

Sleep and Stress Management for a Flat Tummy: The Role of Rest and Relaxation

This chapter will discuss the importance of sleep and stress management for achieving a flat tummy. Many people need to realize the impact of sleep and stress on their weight and overall health.

Lack of sleep and chronic stress can increase the hormone cortisol, promoting the accumulation of belly fat. Additionally, lack of sleep can lead to cravings for unhealthy foods and decreased physical activity levels.

Here are some tips for improving your sleep and stress management to support a flatter tummy:

1. Prioritize sleep:

Aim for at least 7-8 hours of sleep per night. Create a relaxing bedtime routine, such as taking a warm bath, reading a book, or meditating, to help you wind down and prepare for sleep. Also, create a sleep-conducive environment, such as keeping your bedroom cool, dark, and quiet.

2. Practice stress-reducing activities:

Incorporate stress-reducing activities into your daily routine, such as yoga, meditation, or deep breathing exercises. These activities can help you manage your stress levels and decrease cortisol production.

3. Get regular physical activity:

Stress levels can be reduced and sleep quality can be improved through regular exercise. Aim for at least 30 minutes of moderate-intensity daily routine, such as brisk walking, cycling, or swimming.

4. *Limit caffeine and alcohol intake:*

Caffeine and alcohol can disrupt sleep patterns and increase stress levels. Don't take these substances before bed, especially if you have trouble sleeping.

5. *Seek support:*

If you're struggling with chronic stress or sleep issues, consider seeking support from a healthcare professional or therapist. They can help you identify the root causes of your stress and develop a plan to manage it more effectively.

By prioritizing sleep and stress management, you can support your body's natural weight management processes and achieve a flatter tummy. Remember, listening to your body and adjusting your routine as needed to support your health and wellness goals is essential.

You can support your body's natural weight management processes and achieve optimal health and wellness by prioritizing sleep, incorporating stress-reducing activities into your routine, getting regular physical activity, limiting caffeine and alcohol intake, and seeking support as needed,

In conclusion, sleep and stress management are essential to a healthy lifestyle and can support your efforts to achieve a flatter tummy.

Chapter 6

The Role of Nutrition in Achieving a Flat Tummy

In addition to exercise, nutrition is crucial in achieving and maintaining a flat tummy. In this chapter, we'll explore the importance of nutrition for weight loss and provide some tips for improving your eating habits.

The Importance of Nutrition for Weight Loss

While exercise is integral to any weight loss plan, what you eat can significantly impact your success. To lose weight, including belly fat, you must create a calorie deficit, which means consuming fewer calories than you burn. This can be achieved by reducing your intake of high-calorie, unhealthy foods and increasing your intake of nutrient-dense, low-calorie foods.

In addition to calorie intake, the types of foods you eat can also affect your weight loss efforts. For example, foods high in protein, fiber, and healthy fats can help keep you full and satisfied, making it easier to stick to your diet.

On the other hand, foods high in refined sugars and unhealthy fats can contribute to weight gain and make it harder to lose weight, including belly fat.

Tips for Improving Your Eating Habits

To get the most out of your nutrition plan and support your weight loss efforts, try incorporating the following tips:

- ***Eat a variety of nutrient-dense foods:***

Aim to consume various of nutrient-dense foods, such as vegetables, fruits, whole grains, lean proteins, and healthy fats, to ensure you get all the nutrients your body needs.

- ***Avoid processed and refined foods:***

To support your weight loss efforts, limit your intake of processed and refined foods, such as fast food, snack foods, and sugary drinks, often high in calories and unhealthy ingredients.

- ***Portion control:***

Pay attention to portion sizes and aim to eat appropriate amounts of food to support your weight loss goals.

- ***Drink plenty of water:***

Water is essential for good health and can help keep you full and satisfied, making it easier to stick to your diet. Aim to drink at least eight cups of water per day.

- ***Eat mindfully:***

Pay attention to what you're eating and try to savor your food rather than eating quickly or on the go. Eating can help you to be more mindful of your food choices and make healthier decisions.

By paying attention to your nutrition and improving your eating habits, you'll be well on your way to achieving a flat tummy.

The Power of Mindfulness and Stress Management for a Flat Tummy

Mindfulness and stress management can play a significant role in achieving and maintaining a flat tummy. Stress and unhealthy coping mechanisms, such as emotional eating, can contribute to weight gain and make it harder to lose weight, including belly fat.

On the other hand, mindfulness and healthy stress management techniques can help to support weight loss efforts and improve overall well-being.

One of the primary benefits of mindfulness for weight loss is its ability to help you become more aware of your thoughts, feelings, and behaviors related to food and exercise.

Practicing mindfulness allows you to tune in to your body's hunger and satiety cues and make healthier food choices. In addition, mindfulness can help reduce stress and improve sleep, which can be factored into weight gain and difficulty losing weight, including belly fat.

To get the most out of mindfulness and stress management for a flat tummy, consider incorporating the following techniques into your routine:

- ***Practice mindfulness meditation:***

Mindfulness meditation involves focusing on the present moment and letting go of judgment. Practicing mindful meditation can help you to become more aware of your thoughts and feelings and develop healthier habits.

- ***Eat mindfully:***

Practice mindfulness while eating by focusing on your food and paying attention to your body's hunger and satiety cues.

- ***Exercise regularly:***

Regular physical activity, such as yoga or walking, can help to reduce stress and improve overall well-being.

- ***Find healthy ways to cope with stress:***

Rather than turning to food or unhealthy behaviors to cope with stress, try finding healthy ways to manage stress, such as talking to a friend, practicing yoga, or walking.

- ***Get enough sleep:***

Adequate sleep is essential for good health and can also help to reduce stress. It is recommended that you sleep between 7-9 hours per night.

By incorporating mindfulness and healthy stress management techniques into your routine, you'll be well on your way to achieving a flat tummy and overall good health.

Supplements for a Flat Tummy: Natural Remedies and Boosters

In this section, we'll discuss supplements' role in achieving a flat tummy. While a healthy diet and regular exercise are the foundation of any weight management plan, natural supplements can also support a leaner midsection. If you're looking to supplement your work-out routine, here are a few suggestions:

1. *Probiotics:*

Gut health can be improved with probiotics, which are live bacteria and yeasts that are beneficial to the gut. Probiotics can support a flatter tummy by promoting healthy digestion and reducing inflammation in the gut.

Look for probiotic supplements that contain a mix of different strains to support overall gut health.

2. Digestive enzymes:

Digestive enzymes aid in the breakdown of food molecules into smaller ones that the body can absorb and utilise for energy. Digestive enzymes can support a flatter tummy by improving digestion and reducing bloating.

Look for digestive enzyme supplements that contain a mix of different enzymes, such as amylase, protease, and lipase.

3. Fiber:

Fiber is a carbohydrate that the body is unable to digest. By promoting healthy digestion and regulating blood sugar levels, fiber can support a flatter tummy.

Look for supplements containing soluble fiber, such as psyllium husk or glucomannan, to help you feel fuller for longer.

4. Green tea extract:

Green tea extract is a natural supplement that contains powerful antioxidants called catechins. By boosting metabolism and reducing inflammation in the body, green tea extract can support a flatter tummy.

Look for supplements that contain at least 50% EGCG, the most potent catechin in green tea.

5. Magnesium:

Magnesium is a mineral that plays a critical role in over 300 biochemical reactions, including regulating blood sugar levels and supporting a healthy metabolism. Magnesium can support a flatter tummy by promoting healthy digestion and reducing inflammation.

Look for supplements containing magnesium citrate or glycinate and two highly absorbable forms of magnesium.

While supplements can support a flatter tummy, it's important to remember that they should not replace a healthy diet and regular exercise. Always talk to your healthcare provider before starting any new supplement regimen, especially if you are pregnant, nursing, or taking medication.

Always prioritize a healthy diet and regular exercise, and consult with your healthcare provider before starting any new supplement regimen.

In conclusion, natural supplements can offer a boost in supporting a leaner midsection. Probiotics, digestive enzymes, fiber, green tea extract, and magnesium are all supplements to consider adding to your routine.

Chapter 7

Flat Tummy-Friendly Lifestyle Habits to Adopt

In addition to exercise and nutrition, adopting certain lifestyle habits can support your efforts to achieve and maintain a flat tummy. Here are some flat tummy-friendly lifestyle habits to consider incorporating into your routine:

1. ***Stay hydrated:***

Drinking enough water can help flush out toxins, support digestion, and keep you full and satisfied, supporting weight loss efforts. Aim to drink at least eight cups of water per day.

2. ***Get enough sleep:***

Adequate sleep is essential for good health and supports weight loss efforts.

3. ***Eat regularly:***

Skipping meals or going long periods without eating can disrupt your metabolism and make it harder to lose weight, including belly fat. Aim to eat regular, balanced meals to support your weight loss efforts.

4. ***Manage stress:***

Stress and unhealthy coping mechanisms, such as emotional eating, can contribute to weight gain and make it harder to lose weight, including belly fat. Find healthy ways to manage stress, such as talking to a friend, practicing yoga, or walking.

5. *Limit alcohol consumption:*

Alcohol can be high in calories and disrupt sleep and increase appetite, making it harder to lose weight, including belly fat. If you do choose to drink alcohol, aim to limit your intake and choose low-calorie options.

6. *Incorporate strength training:*

In addition to cardio, strength training is an integral part of any weight loss plan, including achieving a flat tummy. Strength training exercises, such as weight lifting and bodyweight exercises, can be practical for burning belly fat because they build muscle, which can increase your metabolism and help you burn more calories throughout the day.

By adopting these flat tummy-friendly lifestyle habits, you'll be well on your way to achieving and maintaining a strong, toned, flat tummy.

Common Mistakes to Avoid on Your Flat Tummy Journey

While working towards a flat tummy can be rewarding, inevitable mistakes can sabotage your efforts and make it harder to achieve your goals. Here are some common mistakes to avoid on your flat tummy journey:

1. ***Skipping meals:***

Skipping meals or going long periods without eating can disrupt your metabolism and make it harder to lose weight, including belly fat. Aim to eat regular, balanced meals to support your weight loss efforts.

2. ***Relying solely on cardio:***

While cardio is an integral part of any weight loss plan, it's also important to incorporate strength training into your routine. Strength training exercises, such as weight lifting and bodyweight exercises, can be practical for burning belly fat because they build muscle, which can increase your metabolism and help you burn more calories throughout the day.

3. **Focusing on quick fixes:**

Fad diets and quick fixes may promise rapid weight loss, but they are often unsustainable and can negatively impact your health. Instead of focusing on quick fixes, make sustainable lifestyle changes supporting weight loss and overall health.

4. **Underestimating the role of nutrition:**

While exercise is an essential part of any weight loss plan, what you eat can significantly impact your success. To lose weight, including belly fat, you must create a calorie deficit, which means consuming fewer calories than you burn.

This can be achieved by reducing your intake of high-calorie, unhealthy foods and increasing your intake of nutrient-dense, low-calorie foods.

By avoiding these common mistakes and focusing on sustainable lifestyle changes, you'll be well on your way to achieving and maintaining a flat tummy.

Healthy Habits for a Flat Tummy: Lifestyle Changes and Daily Practices

This section will discuss the healthy habits you can adopt to support a flatter tummy. While diet and exercise are essential in achieving a leaner midsection, healthy habits and daily practices can also make a big difference.

Here are some healthy habits to consider adding to your routine:

1. ***Stay hydrated:***

Drinking water throughout the day can help support healthy digestion and reduce bloating.

Aim to drink at least eight glasses of water per day and avoid sugary drinks that can lead to inflammation in the body.

2. *Practice mindful eating:*

Mindful eating is the practice of being present and fully engaged with the experience of eating. It involves paying attention to your body's natural signals of hunger and fullness, and intentionally eating at a slower pace. By practicing mindful eating, you can reduce overeating and support healthy digestion.

3. *Manage stress:*

Chronic stress can lead to inflammation in the body and contribute to weight gain. Incorporating stress-reducing practices such as yoga, meditation, or deep breathing exercises can help support a flatter tummy.

4. Get enough sleep:

Adequate sleep is crucial for weight management and overall health. Lack of sleep can increase appetite, cravings for unhealthy foods, and decrease metabolism. Aim for at least 7-8 hours of sleep per night to support a flatter tummy.

5. Move your body:

Regular physical activity can help burn calories and support healthy weight management. Add at least 30 minutes of moderate-intensity exercises, such as brisk walking or cycling, into your daily routine.

6. Limit alcohol intake:

Alcohol can lead to inflammation in the body and contribute to weight gain, especially in the midsection. Limit your alcohol intake and choose lower-calorie options such as light beer or wine.

7. *Practice good posture:*

Good posture can help engage your core muscles and support a flatter tummy. Practice sitting and standing up straight, and avoid slouching or hunching over.

In conclusion, adopting healthy habits and daily practices can support a flatter tummy in addition to a healthy diet and regular exercise. Staying hydrated, practicing mindful eating, managing stress, getting enough sleep, moving your body, limiting alcohol intake, and practicing good posture are all habits to consider incorporating into your routine.

Remember that small changes can make a big difference, and prioritize consistency and self-care in your weight management journey.

In the next chapter, we'll examine the different ways of staying motivated and remaining on track with your goals while trying to achieve and maintain a flat tummy.

Chapter 8

Staying Motivated and On Track with Your Goals

Staying motivated and on track with your flat tummy goals can be challenging, especially when faced with setbacks or obstacles. Here are vital tips for staying motivated and on track with your goals:

1. **Set specific, achievable goals:**

Rather than setting vague goals, such as "I want to lose weight," set specific, achievable goals that are measurable and time-bound. For example, "As long as I eat a healthy, balanced diet and exercise three times a week, I will lose 10 pounds in three months."

2. ***Keep a journal:***

Keeping a journal can be a helpful way to track your progress and stay motivated. In your journal, you can write down your goals, what you're doing to achieve them, and any challenges or setbacks you encounter.

3. ***Find a support system:***

A support system, whether it's a group of friends, a fitness coach, or a supportive partner, can help keep you motivated and accountable.

4. ***Celebrate small victories:***

It's important to celebrate your progress, no matter how small. Celebrating small wins can motivate you to continue working towards your goals.

5. **Be kind to yourself:**

It's important to be kind to yourself and not get discouraged by setbacks or obstacles. Remember that progress takes time, and it's okay to make mistakes along the way.

By setting specific, achievable goals, tracking your progress, finding a support system, celebrating your victories, and being kind to yourself, you'll be well on your way to staying motivated and on track with your flat tummy goals.

The Role of Supplements in Achieving a Flat Tummy

While diet and exercise are essential to achieving and maintaining a flat tummy, supplements can also support weight loss efforts. However, it's vital to know that supplements do not replace a healthy diet and exercise program and should be used with a well-rounded lifestyle. Here is some information about the role of supplements in achieving a flat tummy:

1. Protein supplements

The nutrient protein plays an essential role in the building and repair of muscles, as well as in maintaining filling and satisfied feelings. Protein supplements, such as whey protein, can be a convenient way to increase your protein intake, particularly if you're having trouble meeting your protein needs through diet alone.

However, it's essential to remember that protein supplements are not a replacement for whole foods and should be used in addition to a healthy diet.

2. Fiber supplements

Fiber is a type of carbohydrate found in plant-based foods, and it can help keep you feeling full and satisfied, which can support weight loss efforts. Some people may have trouble getting enough fiber in their diet, and fiber supplements, such as psyllium husk or glucomannan, can be a convenient way to increase fiber intake.

However, it's essential to speak with a healthcare professional before starting any fiber supplement, as they can interfere with certain medications and cause gastrointestinal side effects if not taken correctly.

3. Fat burners

Some supplements, such as thermogenic or fat burners, are marketed to support weight loss and loss, including belly fat. These supplements may contain caffeine, green tea extract, or conjugated linoleic acid (CLA), which boosts metabolism and increase fat burning.

However, it's essential to be aware that the effectiveness of these supplements is often unproven, and they may have potential side effects, such as jitteriness, insomnia, and digestive issues.

In addition, it's essential to remember that these supplements are not a replacement for a healthy diet and exercise program and should be used with a well-rounded lifestyle.

It's also important to know that dietary supplements' quality and safety can vary. Some supplements may be contaminated with harmful ingredients or may not contain the ingredients listed on the label.

To ensure the quality and safety of any supplement, you must purchase from a reputable source and speak with a healthcare professional before starting any supplement regimen.

In summary, while supplements may support weight loss and loss, including belly fat, they are not a replacement for a healthy diet and exercise program and should be used in conjunction with a well-rounded lifestyle.

It's essential to be aware of supplements' potential risks and limitations and to speak with a healthcare professional before starting any supplement regimen.

Beyond the Flat Tummy: Maintaining Your Results and Living a Healthy Lifestyle

Achieving a flat tummy can be a great accomplishment, but the real challenge is maintaining your results and living a healthy lifestyle over the long term. It's easy to fall back into old habits and undo all your hard work, but with the right strategies and mindset, you can go beyond the flat tummy and achieve lasting health and wellness.

1. *Set realistic goals:*

When it comes to maintaining your results, it's essential to set realistic goals that are achievable and sustainable. Setting realistic goals might mean shifting your focus from the number on the scale to how you feel in your body or setting goals that focus on health and wellness rather than just appearance.

2. *Keep track of your progress:*

It can be very helpful to monitor your progress so that you remain motivated and stay on track. You might keep track of your progress by:

- Taking photos.
- Keeping a food and exercise journal.

- Using a fitness tracker to track your steps and activity levels.

3. Focus on sustainable habits:

Rather than following a strict diet or workout plan, focus on building sustainable habits you can maintain over the long term. Focusing on sustainable habits might mean incorporating more whole foods into your diet, finding activities you enjoy that get you moving, and practicing stress-management techniques that work for you.

4. Find a support system:

A support system can make all the difference in maintaining your results and staying motivated. Finding a support system might include the following:

- Joining a fitness community.

- Finding a workout buddy.
- Working with a health coach or therapist to help you stay on track.

5. *Celebrate your successes:*

Celebrating your successes along the way is essential, no matter how small they may seem. Celebrating accomplishments can motivate you and remind you how far you've come. Treat yourself to a massage, buy a new workout outfit, or take a moment to reflect on your progress and pat yourself on the back.

In conclusion, going beyond the flat tummy requires a holistic approach to health and wellness. By setting realistic goals, tracking your progress, focusing on sustainable habits, finding a support system, and celebrating your successes, you can maintain your results and live a healthy, fulfilling life for years.

Chapter 9

Celebrating Your Success and Maintaining a Flat Tummy for Life

Congratulations on completing your journey towards a flat tummy! Achieving and maintaining a flat tummy requires dedication, hard work, and commitment to a healthy lifestyle.

By incorporating regular exercise, a healthy diet, mindfulness and stress management techniques, and flat tummy-friendly lifestyle habits into your routine, you've taken important steps towards achieving and maintaining a strong, toned, and flat tummy.

As you celebrate your success, it's important to remember that maintaining a flat tummy is a lifelong journey. To maintain your results, it's important to continue making healthy lifestyle choices and to be mindful of your habits. Here are some tips for maintaining a flat tummy for life:

1. **Continue exercising regularly:**

Regular physical activity is essential for good health and maintaining a flat tummy. Aim to incorporate a mix of cardio and strength training into your exercise routine to support muscle building and fat burning.

2. **Eat a balanced, nutritious diet:**

A healthy diet is an important foundation for maintaining a flat tummy. Aim to consume a variety of nutrient-dense foods, such as vegetables, fruits, whole grains, lean proteins, and healthy fats, to ensure that you're getting all of the nutrients your body needs.

3. **Manage stress:**

Stress and unhealthy coping mechanisms, such as emotional eating, can contribute to weight gain and make it harder to maintain a flat tummy. Find healthy ways to manage stress, such as talking to a friend, practicing yoga, or taking a walk.

4. **Stay hydrated:**

Drinking enough water can help to flush out toxins, support digestion, and keep you feeling full and satisfied, which can support weight loss and maintenance efforts. Aim to drink at least eight cups of water per day.

5. **Get enough sleep:**

Adequate sleep is essential for good health and can also support weight maintenance efforts. Aim for 7-9 hours of sleep per night.

By continuing to make healthy lifestyle choices and being mindful of your habits, you'll be well on your way to maintaining a flat tummy for life. Don't forget to celebrate your success and reward yourself for all of the hard work you've put in. You deserve it!

Conclusion

Congratulations on completing this book and taking the first step towards achieving a flat tummy and a healthier lifestyle. By now, you should have a solid understanding of the science behind a leaner midsection, the best nutrition strategies for a flat tummy, the importance of mindset and motivation, sleep and stress management, and the benefits of supplements and healthy habits.

It's time to put your knowledge into action and start implementing the strategies outlined in this book. Remember, achieving a flat tummy is not a quick fix or a one-size-fits-all solution. It requires commitment, patience, and a willingness to make sustainable lifestyle changes that work for you and your body.

Here are some action steps you can take to get started:

1. ***Create a plan***: Use the strategies outlined in this book to create a plan that works for you. Creating a might include setting realistic goals, creating a meal plan, finding an exercise routine you enjoy, and incorporating stress-management techniques into your daily routine.

2. ***Stay accountable***: Find a way to stay accountable to your goals, whether by tracking your progress, working with a coach or accountability partner, or joining a fitness community.

3. ***Be patient***: Remember that achieving a flat tummy and a healthier lifestyle is a journey, not a destination. Seeing results takes time and consistency, so be patient and trust the process.

4. ***Celebrate your successes***: Take the time to celebrate them along the way, no matter how small they may seem. Celebrating your accomplishments will help keep you

motivated and remind you how far you've come.

5. ***Keep learning***: The science of health and wellness constantly evolves, so stay curious and keep learning. Continuously educate yourself on the latest research and best practices, and be open to trying new strategies that may work for you.

In conclusion, achieving a flat tummy and a healthier lifestyle is a journey that requires commitment, patience, and a willingness to make sustainable lifestyle changes. By following the strategies outlined in this book and taking action, you can achieve your goals and live a happier, healthier life. Good luck on your journey!

Thank you for choosing "*The Flat Tummy Blueprint*". We hope that it has been helpful and that you feel empowered to continue on your journey towards a healthy and strong body.

About the Author

Kayla S. Brigman is a certified health professional, personal trainer and nutritionist with over 16 years of experience helping clients achieve their fitness goals. Her passion for fitness began at a young age and has led her to work with a variety of clients, from professional athletes to busy moms. She believes that everyone can achieve their ideal body with the right tools and mindset.

In addition to her work as a trainer and nutritionist, Kayla is also a writer and speaker on topics related to health and wellness. Her articles have been featured in several fitness publications and she has spoken at conferences and events.

Kayla is committed to helping others live their best lives through fitness and nutrition.

Other Books by the Author

Below are other amazing book(s) by Kayla S. Brigman

BOOK TITLE	BOOK COVER	LINK TO READ
End The Snore Struggle		Click Here to read for free on Kindle Unlimited
The Art of Being Fresh		Click Here to read for free on Kindle Unlimited

The Lean Body Blueprint	THE LEAN BODY BLUEPRINT — A STEP-BY-STEP GUIDE TO LOSING FAT BUILDING MUSCLE — KAYLA S BRIGMAN	<u>Click Here to read for free on Kindle Unlimited</u>
Postpartum Body Rejuvenation For Women	POSTPARTUM BODY REJUVENATION FOR WOMEN — KAYLA S. BRIGMAN	<u>Click Here to read for free on Kindle Unlimited</u>
Kiss Bad Breath Goodbye	KISS BAD BREATH GOODBYE — THE ULTIMATE GUIDE TO ELIMINATING MOUTH ODOR — KAYLA S. BRIGMAN	<u>Click Here to read for free on Kindle Unlimited</u>

The Anti-Aging Blueprint	THE ANTI-AGING BLUEPRINT KAYLA S. BRIGMAN	[Click Here to read for free on Kindle Unlimited](#)
Going Bald with Grace	GOING BALD WITH GRACE Embracing and Empowering Yourself after Hair Loss KAYLA S. BRIGMAN	[Click Here to read for free on Kindle Unlimited](#)

THE END